Sunflower Spirit

26 Ways to Follow the Light of Self, Others, and Spirit While Journeying with Cancer

Anne Marie Bennett

Dedication

This book is for the worldwide SoulCollage® community:
You surrounded me on my second cancer journey
with unconditional love, sweet prayer and divine healing intention
from all corners of the world.
I have truly learned and absorbed
the healing power of community
from all of you.
Thank you. Thank you.

Introduction

Greetings! I am delighted that you have chosen to ease the burden of cancer in your life, and to shine the light of S.O.S. (Self, Others and Spirit) upon your journey by reading and using this workbook.

Each of the 26 sections here acts as a stand-alone idea or experience. My best suggestion is for you to read through the Table of Contents and pay close attention on the inside to which chapters are calling for your attention. Start there. If they are ALL calling your name, start at the beginning and skim through all the pages. When you get to an exercise that appeals to you, set the book aside for a few days or weeks and allow yourself to really experience the activity. Go as deep as you can with whichever ideas call to you.

Living a life with cancer as a constant companion is not easy, nor is it simple. It can be a dark, lonely, frightening journey. My hope in offering this book to you is that it will be a counter-companion to your travels with cancer. Instead of giving in to the fear, may you find a bright and meaningful connection with the Divine. Instead of isolating from others, may you be blessed with the bright light of your personal Community. And instead of running away from feelings and disturbing thoughts, may you find sanctuary within your own brilliant, authentic Self.

I have chosen Sunflower Spirit as the title of this book because of the scene in the movie *Calendar Girls* where the husband takes his wife out to a beautiful field of sunflowers and tells her this:

I don't think there's anything on this planet that more trumpets life than the sunflower. For me that's because of the reason behind its name. Not because it looks like the sun but because it **follows** *the sun. During the course of the day, the head tracks the journey of the sun across the sky. A satellite dish for sunshine. Wherever light is, no matter how weak, these flowers will find it. And that's such an admirable thing. And such a lesson in life.*

This is my hope for you, dear reader. As you read this book, may you continue to follow the light of Self, Others, and Spirit.

Blessings on your journey,

Anne Marie Bennett
Beverly, MA
December 2013

Many hours and much creative energy
were devoted to the creation of this workbook.
Your purchase supports the continuing efforts of *SOS Cancer Journeys*
in its mission to make spiritual/emotional
support and community available
to women with cancer around the world.
To give feedback or to contact the author,
please email annemarie@sos-cancer-journeys.com

This book is brought to you by

SOS Cancer Journeys

*Creatively Connecting Women with Cancer
to Self, Others, and Spirit*
www.sos-cancer-journeys.com

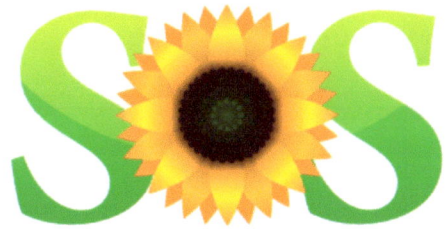

Connecting women with cancer to Self, Others, & Spirit

Table of Contents

A is for... Anchors

Okay, you've been diagnosed with the dreaded C word- Cancer. Or you're already in the middle of treatment. Or maybe you're even *out* of treatment and trying to find your way back out of the maze of doctors' visits, blood tests, and too many trips to the bathroom. What can you do to ground yourself, to remember to come home to yourself in the midst of the dizzying array that sometimes defines us as cancer patients? What can you do? Give yourself some anchors!

I'm not talking about a 500 pound iron boat mooring, although what you'll use will secure you to your own beautiful soul just as tightly. I'm talking about choosing four words that you can repeat, say, hum, drum, or sing over and over (and over again) to yourself whenever you feel yourself coming untethered.

After I was diagnosed with secondary angiosarcoma (left breast), my breast surgeon sent me for a PET scan. I was very afraid, not of the actual test, but of what the test might show. I brought my iPod with me, and a book, but the technician told me I had to sit in a darkened room, in the quiet, and be very still while I drank the two bottles of milky liquid. No music, no books. Huh? I was preparing to distract myself, but instead, I had to sit in darkened silence. I now count this as a major blessing.

In the hushed stillness of that tiny room with the comfy recliner, I let my thoughts wander… and in the meanderings of my mind was a determination that I had not noticed before. I decided right then and there that I was going to get through this, that I wanted to live, was choosing to live. And with that decision, I also chose four words: Breath, Gratitude, Kindness, Joy. Throughout my cancer journey, and even now, I still return to this seven-syllable mantra that inevitably reminds me to focus on what *really* matters. Repeating this incantation always serves to anchor me to who I *really* am, what is *most* important to me, and moves me *away from* identifying myself only as a "cancer patient.

You Try It! ~ 4 Little Words

Spend a day or two thinking about what is most important to you in your life right now. What four words will *you* choose to use as anchors that will keep you tethered to your own beautiful soul? Here are some ideas to try out. Roll them over on your tongue, test them out in your heart... which ones resonate? Circle the ones you are immediately drawn to, and then spend some time with them, and narrow it down from there. If you don't like the idea of choosing *four* anchors, it's perfectly okay to choose two or three. Any more than four, though, and you might lose focus.

Peace   Silence   Breath   Wisdom   Heart

Kindness   Joy   Gratitude   Ease   Comfort

Creativity   Stillness   Wonder   Love   Simplicity

Possibility   Angels   Acceptance   Shine

Beauty   Freedom   Boundaries   Light   Patience

Abundance   Community   Divine   Spirit   Enough   Flow

Fearless   Mother Earth   Gentleness   Hope   Laughter   Vision

Forgiveness   Nourishment   Passion   Worthy   Sacred   Whole

Radiance   Receive   Solitude

Don't spend more than a few days deciding! You can always change them later. It's most important that you choose four that resonate with you now and start using them, repeatedly, as you go through your days, your treatments, any tests/procedures that you need to have, or surgery recovery.

B is for... Brighter Thoughts

The primary cause of unhappiness is never the situation but your thoughts about it. Be aware of the thoughts you are thinking. Separate them from the situation, which is always neutral, which always is as it is. – Eckhart Tolle

When I wrote my book about my first journey with cancer (2002), I called it *Bright Side of the Road*, because it seemed like the biggest lesson I took with me from that year of surgeries and treatments was the fact that I actually can *choose* the thoughts that float through my mind. Well, maybe I can't always choose the actual *thoughts*, but what I *can* do is change the *direction* they take. I can choose to latch on to a difficult, negative thought and let it drag me down into the murky swamps of harmful thinking. OR... I can become aware of it, and then choose to let it go. At any given moment, I am at choice.

When I was about to have my first lumpectomy, my surgeon called me to say that the date had to be postponed because of his vacation. At first I was angry, frustrated, and very upset. I had to wait *another week*. What if the cancer cells "caught hold" of me in that span of time and started to "travel" before he could operate on me and take out the lump?

I could hear myself spinning out of control, and I could feel the havoc that these fearful thoughts were wreaking on my quest for inner peace. So I decided that I would choose a *brighter* thought that brought me more comfort and ease: *I'm glad that my surgeon is going on vacation the week before he operates on me, because he'll be well rested and better able to focus on my surgery when he gets back. I'm glad I have a surgeon who takes vacations and isn't overworked and overtired!* With that conscious switch in my mind, I was able to breathe more deeply and actually relax, instead of giving in to the fearful thoughts of the cancer spreading.

You might be shaking your head and thinking that all this emphasis on "bright thoughts" is in complete denial of any anger, fear, grief or frustration you are feeling. Not so! Skip ahead to *F is for... Feelings*. You'll see what I mean!

You Try It! ~ Affirmations

Vivian Green once said, "It is not our circumstances that create our discontent or contentment. It is US." I'm going out on a limb here and saying that this is absolutely true, even in the case of being diagnosed with cancer. It is possible to catch negative thoughts and transform them… which in turn transforms *us* and the way we approach our journey.

This week, pay attention to the thoughts that run screaming through your mind. Notice which ones make you fear-full, and which ones bring you comfort and ease. The next time a Fear-Quaking Thought rumbles through you, catch it! Then transform it into a brighter statement. These brighter thoughts are called affirmations.

You can write a few of your own affirmations, based on whatever Fear-Quaking Thoughts are attacking you. Copy them onto index cards or print them out on little slips of colored paper and post them around your living space where you will see them often- your mirror, the kitchen cupboard, the car's dashboard, your bureau.

Here are some examples:

Fear-Quaking Thought	**Brighter Thought/Affirmation**
I can't get through this.	I CAN get through this.
No one else will love me again.	I am capable of loving and being loved.
The cancer might return.	Just for today, I am safe.
I shouldn't be feeling this way.	All of my feelings are normal.
I hate being bald.	I'm saving money on hair maintenance!

Let it become a game. Take anything that is difficult about your cancer journey, accept it, and talk about it until you feel clear. Then (and only then) add on "The good thing is…." and see what pops out of you!

C is for... Creativity

There are three things you might be thinking right now:

1. I'm not creative. Not me. Never have been.
2. What is she talking about? I have no idea what this has to do with cancer.
3. I *am* a creative woman. Let the fun begin!

If you are in the #3 camp, you have permission to skip this page and move on to the "You Try It" section that follows. Enjoy! Are you thinking more along the lines of #1 or #2? Then read on, dear one, read on.

I am a firm believer in the fact that everyone is creative. Yes, *everyone*! If you've been to one of my websites, you've probably seen a great deal of evidence of my creativity. Collages galore. Color everywhere. A couple of expressive books. Beautiful, informative (let's hope!) online communities. And hey, even my suit-wearing, briefcase-carrying accountant of a husband is creative. Sure, he doesn't paint or make greeting cards or write books, but he is constantly creating positive and money-saving solutions for his clients. He has created a loving family and a home that people love to visit (okay, I helped him with that part!).

Creativity reveals itself in peoples' lives in many ways. When I say "You are a creative woman," that doesn't necessarily mean that you can draw or paint. Here are some ways that creativity might express itself in your life: gardening, cooking, baking, creating comfortable living spaces, creating order from chaos, graphic designing, writing, daydreaming, doodling, gathering people together, planning parties, singing, acting, writing poetry, business development, meeting planning. *You* decide what else!

During both of my Cancer Journeys (2002 and 2011-12), I was often too tired to do creative things. But on my good days, I found great pleasure in making SoulCollage® cards, gathering images, doodling in my art journal, and creating healthy images of myself in my imagination.

You Try It! ~ SOS Collage

How are YOU creative? Make a list and keep it nearby to remind you that you have other passions besides visiting the hospital every week (or every day) for some kind of healing treatments. When you discover that you have a little more energy, go ahead and get out the knitting or embroidery, sing a song in the shower, glue together a little collage and hang it on your wall. Make something new!

Here's another idea. Take the "SOS" outlined letters on the next page, and re-create them on a huge sheet of paper or poster board.   Remember what the letters stand for:

S- Self
O- Others
S- Spirit

Create a collage within the confines of each letter that expresses, for you, the meaning of each word.

For example, in the first S you might glue magazine images that remind you of your real self: people doing things you love to do, or anything that expresses your authentic self.

In the O, you could glue photos (or copies of photos) of people you love, your family and friends, doctors, nurses, and anyone who truly cares about you who is helping you on this cancer journey. Be sure to include people you may not have met, whose inspiration and strength lends you support and courage.   And don't forget your pets!

In the final S, you could glue pictures that give expression to your relationship with Spirit, however you choose to define Spirit.

If this feels too difficult right now, you can just color in the letters with crayons (yes, crayons!) or colored pencils. Print the page out several times and doodle your heart out. Take one with you to the hospital on a treatment day and allow the coloring to soothe and relax you. You can always make a bigger collage another day (or month!).

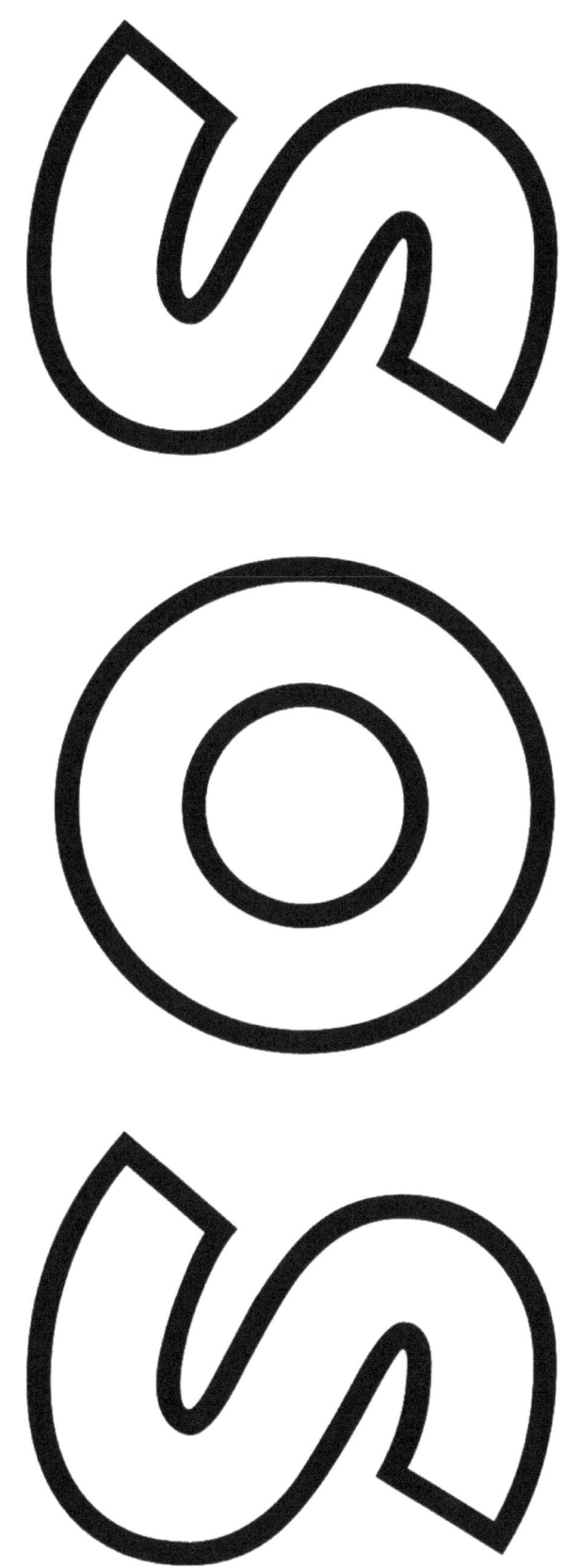

D is for...

Divine Connection

I clearly remember a dark winter morning in December of 2001. My husband was driving me to the hospital where I was to have a stereotactic biopsy. Just whispering the name of this test brought fear into my bones. I was flipping through the current issue of *Real Simple* magazine in the car that morning as my husband negotiated traffic, and I came across an article by Lindsey Crittenden, called "How to Pray." I don't remember much else about the article, except for this prayer that she suggested as a way to begin:

God, You are here.
God, I am here.

I clung to that prayer throughout that morning like a child clings to a soft beloved blanket. And it brought me a deeper security than I had up until then experienced in regards to the fact that I might or might not be embarking on a journey with cancer.

That dark December morning was the first time I had truly reached out to the Divine in many years. As a child, teenager and young adult, I was drawn to Spirit, and to spiritual people and things. As an adult I had been very active in three different Episcopal churches, but during the years preceding this ugly-sounding biopsy, I had isolated myself from church, and from God (whom I now choose to call Spirit). There are many reasons for this, and I find that none of them are relevant right now. What matters is that I came across that article at just the right time. What matters is that I took comfort in those words: *God, You are here. God, I am here.*

Throughout both of my journeys with cancer, one of the greatest lessons I have learned is that I am not alone. There is a divine energy that is larger, more powerful, and more loving than we can possibly imagine. No matter what you call it, it is constantly ready to offer love, guidance, shelter, comfort and wisdom.

You Try It! ~ A Simple Prayer

Find a way to reach out to the Divine, however you choose to call the Divine. Here are some names you might choose to use:

God　　　Spirit　　　　Source　　　The One Buddha Jesus　　　　Divine

Jehovah　　All in All　　Goddess　Yahweh　　Higher Power　Allah　　Mother Earth

Feel free to add any name that suits your own faith or religion. What matters here is that you are reaching out to a power greater than yourself, and asking for guidance on your journey. Ask for comforting arms to hold you and protect you. Ask for whatever you truly need.

Breathe the words of the prayer below as a mantra, during any time you are waiting for a treatment or doctor appointment. Use it when you first wake up, and before you go to sleep. Close your eyes and feel the presence of Spirit. If you like, change the word "God" in this prayer to any name that feels better to you.

On the in breath: *God, You are here.*
On the out breath: *God, I am here.*

There are many other ways to make divine connection a part of your Cancer Journey. Perhaps you have a religious or spiritual community where you feel close to Spirit. Maybe you feel closer to Spirit when you are out in Nature, or with a grandchild, or while you are journaling. Keep in mind that Spirit is with you, no matter what. Invite Spirit with you to your doctor appointments, surgeries and treatments.

Meditate on or journal with this poem, author unknown:

Who I am is a child of the universe.
My soul has a place that cannot be shaken
by external events.
Rooted in Spirit,
my soul is ever-cherished,
ever-known,
and beloved.

E is for... Expression

Dictionary.com defines "Self-Expression" as: *the expression or assertion of one's own personality, as in conversation, behavior, poetry, or painting.* Now, for any of you who are panicking about those words "poetry, or painting," please don't worry! Let's just focus on self-expression in terms of conversation and behavior (for now).

I can't emphasize strongly enough how vital this is. Finding ways to express yourself is important enough on a regular life journey, but when you're traveling for a while with cancer, it becomes an essential tool for the road.

We're talking about expressing feelings here, of course. Let's face it, if you're feeling sad and you don't express that sadness, it's probably going to burrow its way into your body and manifest later on as some kind of physical ailment. The same goes for anger, grief, fear, guilt, shame and frustration.

You can express feelings in several ways. For me, the most helpful thing is writing it all down, but you might be more of a talker, or a mover. You might find it helpful to shut the door of your car, roll up the windows and vent your anger by singing out loud (I mean *screaming* loud) to a heavy metal rock song. Or you might want to go home and pound some pillows, chop some wood, or smack a few golf balls. Find a nonjudgmental, caring friend who will hold your hand while you cry.

Maybe words or tears or whacking little white balls just won't cut it. You might find that you can express yourself best by getting out the crayons or colored pencils or paints, and splashing color onto a page (or pages). Whatever it is… find a way to get the feelings *out of your body and into the world*, where they have less power to harm you. There's more coming about this in *F is for…Feelings*, next.

You Try It! ~ Express Yourself

We're also talking about finding some ways to express who you really are, the *beautiful wonderful YOU* that lies beneath all the exterior accouterments of cancer (hospital gowns, scars, medicine, drains, burned skin, bandages…etc).

When I was going through my cancer journeys, I continually felt the urge to have my doctors and nurses see ME as something other than a patient. I was able to do this by the things I brought with me to my chemo treatments, by talking with my radiation techs about a song I liked or a play I had just seen, and by creating a special handmade card for my surgeon. I spent several hours searching online for a cotton fabric that had koi fish on it (my surgeon's last name is Karp), and then finding someone who would sew several surgical caps for him as a gift. As long as I was doing something (or even just thinking about doing something) that was quintessentially ME, my journey felt lighter, easier, brighter.

This doesn't mean you have to bake brownies for your oncologist, or knit a scarf for your chemo nurse. The idea here is just to try to remember that you are a living, breathing woman, and that cancer isn't the only thing that defines you right now.

So go ahead… make a list of what it is that makes YOU essentially YOU. Go back and look at the images you glued onto the first S in the "You Try It" section of *C is for…Creativity*. And then find some ways to incorporate at least one of them into your journey. You don't even have to involve your medical team. You can make this just for beautiful YOU.

Untie your tongue and untwist those knots in your belly. Let your feelings be known and don't hold back. Express yourself. If you're grieving, cry. If you're angry, be so. Use words. Write them down, speak them, put them out for the world to hear. Express yourself. Use crayons, use clay, use your clarinet. Express yourself with your hands. Draw pictures in the dirt, finger paint, knit. Express your feelings for someone else. Write a song. Sing it out loud. Pick out tiny gifts that express your love, your gratitude, your apologies, and send them off in tiny boxes filled with glitter or confetti.

---from *Words of Wisdom for Women*, Rachel Snyder

F is for... Flow of Feelings

Let everything happen to you. Beauty and Terror. Just keep going. No feeling is final. ~ **Rilke**

Okay, I know what you're thinking. Who has time for feelings when you're dealing with cancer? Let's face it, when we receive a cancer diagnosis, it's mostly all about immediate and important medical decisions: *What procedures, surgeries, treatments should I have? Do I need a second opinion? How will I pay for this? What will my boss say about taking time off? How should I tell my family and friends?*

There's really not a lot of time for feelings when you're facing this bombardment of decisions that usually need to be made NOW. And yet... and yet, you have feelings. We all have feelings flowing around inside of us, whether we're sitting on a beach at sunset with our best beloved by our side, standing aboard the Titanic as it's going down, or somewhere in between.

Even amidst the chaos that your life sometimes becomes when you're diagnosed with cancer, it's important to remember that you are *human*, that you have *feelings*, and that you have permission, *permission*, <u>permission</u>, to feel **anything** you are feeling. Give yourself as much time and space as you need to experience and process any anger or fear or sadness or grief or frustration or loneliness or helplessness that is coming up.

Remember also: whatever you are *feeling* determines what you *need*. So try to give yourself a few moments a few times during each day where you simply STOP, and ask yourself *What am I feeling right now?* Then, based on what you feel, come up with one *I need...*statement. Finally, find a way to safely give yourself what you need. For example:

I feel angry. **I need** to hit something.
How will I meet this need? I will go home and punch my pillows for 5 minutes.

I feel scared. **I need** some comfort.
How will I meet this need? I will say a prayer (or sit with my cat, or ask a friend to hold me while I cry).

You Try It! - Feelings Flow

I learned this exercise from the process of EBT (Emotional Brain Training) as taught by Laurel Mellin. It's a powerful thing to do when you become aware of strong feelings coursing through you. It's a form of verbal expression (see pages 15-16) that you can do either in writing or aloud with a trusted partner. The idea is to use each of the eight sentence-starters below, and *keep saying* each one, until the feeling has passed through your body and mind. Then and only then, move on to the next one.

Sometimes there will be many sentences and sometimes only a few. Also, it's important not to skip any one of the 8 feelings. Breathe deeply before you begin. Put your hand over your heart, knowing that it is safe and normal to be feeling *whatever* you are feeling and to be giving voice to these feelings. It's a healthy thing to do this at least once a day. Here's a short example of what this might look like in your journal (and keep in mind that sometimes this can go on for a few pages or more).

I feel angry that I've got cancer AGAIN. I feel angry that I have to go through chemo again. I HATE IT THAT my body did this to me. I feel sad that I'm going to lose my left breast. I feel sad that I have to give that up in order to be free of the cancer. I feel sad that I don't have a choice about this. I feel afraid that this time the cancer is going to kill me. I feel afraid that the surgeon won't get it all out of me. I feel afraid that I'm going to die before I'm ready. I feel afraid that the cancer has already spread. I feel afraid that people are going to look at me differently. I feel guilty for not going to the doctor sooner. I feel guilty for not eating healthy all the time. I feel guilty for snapping at my husband yesterday.

It's really REALLY important that you do let it ALL out, and take as many pages as you need. KEEP THE SENTENCES VERY SHORT. Don't go into explanations of *why* you are feeling this way, or what this doctor said or how that friend treated you. Just keep the **short sentences** flowing. Don't stop to think about what you are writing. This is about the FEELINGS! Be sure that each sentence begins with *I feel…* and do them in the order of the worksheet on the next page.

Once you have the first 4 more difficult feelings (notice I didn't say "bad" or "negative" feelings) out of you, it will be easier to do the other side of the feelings flow.

Feelings Flow Worksheet

I feel angry that…

I feel sad that…

I feel afraid that…

I feel guilty that…

I feel grateful that…

I feel happy that…

I feel secure that…

I feel proud that…

Note: Just use this page as a guideline for this practice, because you probably will need more space!

G is for...

Gratitude

You might be familiar with this because it's a pretty "hot" topic around the world today. I was "practicing gratitude" long before cancer made its way into my life. So when I found myself face to face with cancer, I was brought up a little short. I was thinking, "How am I going to say *thank you* for THIS?" and "How on earth can I possibly be *grateful* for having cancer?"

Well, that turned out to be an important question to ask! And I gently suggest that at some point on your own Cancer Journey, you ask yourself this same question.

Having been down Cancer Avenue twice now in the last decade, I am positively certain that Cancer always comes bearing gifts. It's just a matter of becoming aware of the gifts, of actively seeking the gifts, and of maybe even reframing (a little bit) what the word "gift" actually means.

Ondrea Levine said: *I believe illness is a great teacher…. It's a wonderful teacher if you can surrender and open to it.*

So that's what this chapter is really about. You're becoming willing to open to a new idea about what gift your own Cancer Journey might be bringing you. This gift is probably not going to look like what you think a "gift" should look like. It's not going to be two round-trip tickets to a Caribbean Island, all expenses paid, a week to lie in the sun with your best beloved by your side, sipping pineapple drinks brought to you by a gorgeous servant. The gift is not going to be a brand new laptop computer or even a sparkly new dress for the office holiday party. But it IS going to be something amazing, something beautiful that you couldn't even possibly dream of.

And the key to discovering this gift (these gifts) is the practice of gratitude. The key to discovering the gifts that cancer offers you is being *open* to the fact that there are actually gifts involved!

You Try It! ~ Thank You For...

My job and yours is to gather grace during our chaotic times,
always remembering the universal support system that underlies
any confusion or disruption.

--- Laura Alden Kamm

It took me a while, during my first cancer journey, to realize that amazing things were happening all around me, even while I was suffering the indignities of surgeries and innumerable doctor visits and difficult choices. I was journaling a lot during that time, and I found that I was noticing and keying in on the little details of my journey: a particular nurse whose touch felt like an angel, my oncologist asking me how my spirits were, a casual acquaintance turning into a close friend, or how my cats seemed to surround me on the bed or sofa whenever I most needed comfort.

I found that I actually felt better, more hopeful, when I was noticing things like this, so every night before I fell asleep, I said these short little prayers, in my mind, silently. Many times, I drifted off to sleep on these lists… and they carried me through many a difficult week. I still do this practice to this day (er, night!).

It can work well as a journaling activity also, but for now, just try getting into the habit of saying "Thank you for…" or "Thank you that…" several times as you close your eyes and wend your way towards sleep. For me, I was saying thank you to Spirit, but you can name Spirit whatever you like! It doesn't even matter what you are calling the Being/Energy/Force that you are saying thank you to. What does matter is that you are becoming more and more aware, on a daily, moment-to-moment basis, of all the blessings that are being offered to you in *spite* of (and maybe even *because* of) this journey you are on with cancer.

If the only prayer you ever say in your entire life is thank you,
it will be enough.

--- Meister Eckhart

H is for... Humor

I remember the day of my first cancer diagnosis so clearly. My doctor had called me in the late afternoon while I was still at work. I immediately went into the rest room and sat on the floor, sobbing. Even though my head was spinning, and my heart was pounding with fear, I made it through a few more hours before I headed home to tell my husband. He was strong and steady; he said the exact right thing, "We'll get through this together." I cried copious tears. I felt like I was backed into a corner, helpless, no way out. Cancer. The C word. Me! I couldn't quite believe it.

Later that evening, we sat together on the sofa, looking for something to take our minds off of the last few stressful hours. I had the remote in my hand and I was flipping channels, not focusing on anything much. My attention was caught when I got to the Public TV channel and saw a female Episcopal priest talking in a jaunty English accent. The Episcopal Church had been a major part of my spiritual journey in my adulthood, so my curiosity was aroused. A TV comedy about a woman priest (*Vicar of Dibley*) seemed right up my alley.

In just a matter of seconds my husband and I were actually *laughing wildly* at the antics of this outspoken, hilarious woman and her sparse congregation of characters. About halfway through the show, I thought, "Wait a minute. I'm *laughing*? I was diagnosed with cancer today. Should I really be *laughing*?" But that thought went completely away with the next ridiculous thing the main character said. My husband and I laughed together for the next 30 minutes, and guess what? I felt much better afterwards, and so did he. Our sleep that night was restful and deep.

I decided right then and there, that *yes indeed*, I *should* be laughing, and I chose to seek out laughter as much as I could during the upcoming months of surgeries and treatments.

You Try It! ~ At the Movies

Research shows us time and again that laughter is very healing, not only for the body, but the mind and spirit as well.

It may sound really crazy to you right now, especially if you've just been diagnosed and are full of powerful feelings like anger, fear, and bewilderment. Just trust me on this. As long as you are giving yourself permission to *feel whatever it is you are feeling* (see pages 15-17), then you are ready to inject a little laughter into your cancer journey.

Okay, here's your assignment. Find a movie or a television show that always makes you laugh, no matter how silly or outrageous it is, or how strange it might seem to someone else. This is for YOU, dear one! And now... *watch it.* Now, today, tomorrow, as soon as you possibly can. Watch it more than once, if you have the time. Watch it from beginning to end, with no interruptions. Do not wash the dishes, check email, do a load of laundry, make dinner or go online shopping while you are watching. Just give yourself over to the movie and allow yourself to laugh out loud as much as you want, as hard as you want, for as long as you want. If you have chosen a funny TV show instead of a movie, try to watch several episodes, one right after the other.

Remember to choose movies/shows that make YOU laugh right out loud. Here are some of my favorites: *My Cousin Vinny, The Big Bang Theory, Modern Family, 3rd Rock from the Sun, Lars and the Real Girl.*

Another assignment: Put this quotation in a place where you'll see it often. Allow it to remind you of how healing laughter can be, even when you're on a cancer journey:

And the depth of the laughter! The way it seemed to go so far down inside it scraped the inside bottoms of the feet. No one laughed like that anymore. Nothing seemed funny enough. When his uncle and his guests finished laughing, they'd seemed lighter, clearer; even their activities appeared to be done more gracefully. It was as if the laughing emptied them, and sharing it placed whatever was laughable and unbearable in its proper perspective.

--- Alice Walker

I is for... Imagery

The world behind our eyes is as important as the world in front of our eyes.
~ Caroline Myss

I'd like you to stop reading right now and take a deep breath. Go ahead. These words will still be here when you get back!

Ahhh....There is something about pausing like this that really can shift, well, everything. In doing this, your blood pressure went down a little bit and your central nervous system had a chance to rewind. Even brief pauses like this throughout your day can affect many levels of healing.

Now, let's go back to the quotation at the top of this page. What is it, exactly, this "world in front of our eyes?" It's your daily world, whatever is happening right now for you- doctor appointments, blood draws, fearful check-ups, play dates with grandchildren, chemo treatments, dinners out with loved ones, ugly scars, beautiful sunsets, and everything in between. These are the important aspects of our everyday lives.

And what about the "world behind our eyes?" This is the world that we create, in our imaginations, and in that world we can build castles, invite celebrities and angels to dine with us, and visualize whatever we need that makes us feel good, inside and out.

Let's take a moment right now and do a little exercise with inner imagery. I have adapted this from Mark Nepo's book, *As Far As the Heart Can See.* Close your eyes and tune into your breathing. Imagine a scene from your cancer journey that brought you a sense of fear or any other deep feeling. You might be remembering a flash of anger at the moment of your diagnosis, or the fearful hour before your surgery, or the anxiety you felt before your first chemo or radiation treatment. Enter that scene. See it, hear it, smell it, if possible. And just breathe as you picture it in your mind, knowing that no matter what, you were and are safe.

Now, imagine a setting or event that brings you great joy. Enter that scene and see it, hear it, smell it, taste it, feel it. Really bring it to life inside of you. Spend a little time there. Allow the joy you are feeling to alleviate any fear from the previous experience.

You Try It! ~
Inner Sanctuary

There! You did it! Using imagery to transform your body, mind and spirit can be as simple as taking a quiet moment, and bringing to mind a loving or joyful memory in order to dissipate the immediate effect of fear or anxiety.

Keep in mind that not everyone can "see" things in their mind's eye. Some people are more prone to *hear* sounds when they do this inner imagery work, or even to *feel* things kinesthetically. Others simply have an inner sense of what is happening. You might even want to use magazine images that invoke feelings of peace and love and joy, if that makes the image come alive more easily for you.

One of the most helpful tools that I used during my own cancer journeys was an inner imagery meditation that I wrote called "Inner Sanctuary." I'm going to take you on this magical inner journey through the audio link below.

The purpose of this particular inner imagery is for you to create a safe place inside of you, where you can go on a daily, weekly, or even hourly basis, in order to find your own true center, your own deep home within. I imagined my own Inner Sanctuary as a big cottage right on the ocean's edge. But yours might be a huge tree in a moonlit forest or a cave, an underwater abode, or a dwelling made of stars.

I went to my Inner Sanctuary often during my recovery from all my surgeries, as well as during my chemo treatments. It was most helpful for falling asleep at night in a peaceful, calm state of mind. I still visit my Inner Sanctuary today. This is fluent imagery that meets you wherever you are, and can change according to your needs at any given time.

So go ahead… enter your own Inner Sanctuary, where your deepest heart and soul are alive and waiting for you.

To listen online, click here:

http://www.audioacrobat.com/play/W5595mb4

To download as an mp3 file, click here:

http://amber56.audioacrobat.com/download/KaleidoSoul-Meditation-Inner-Sanctuary.mp3

Inner Sanctuary- Journaling Questions

You might find it helpful to journal with these questions after your first Inner Sanctuary experience. See if you can discover even more things about this special inner place.

1. What does your Inner Sanctuary look like?

2. Describe the setting of your Inner Sanctuary. What is nearby? What surrounds it?

3. How did you feel when you entered this safe place?

4. Describe the interior of your Inner Sanctuary. What do you like most about this space?

5. What does the word refuge mean to you?

6. How can this inner space be a refuge to you while you are on your own cancer journey?

7. What was in the blue velvet box that you found by the door? What did you do with it?

8. Who do you think gave you the gift that was in the blue velvet box?

9. Go back to the Inner Sanctuary again, and pause the recording during the exploring time so that you have more than 90 seconds to explore. Stay there for several minutes. Try doing the Feelings Flow (see page 19) while you are there. What happens next?

10. The beautiful thing about this meditation is that after listening to it several times, you will probably be able to close your eyes and "go there" on your

J is for... Joy!

Anything you have suffered - the moment you wake up it becomes the raw material for joy. ~ Martha Beck

I know that you might be wondering why I'm including a section about Joy in a book about cancer. Let me explain. Joy is not just for healthy people! And contrary to what I learned when I was young, joy is not just to be experienced at Christmas, Easter and birthdays.

I believe that Mark Nepo says it best below. Take a few moments now and read this out loud. Close your eyes and let the words reverberate in your soul.

... the extraordinary is waiting quietly beneath the skin of all that is ordinary. Light is in both the broken bottle and the diamond, and music is in both the flowing violin and the water dripping from the drainage pipe. Yes, God is under the porch as well as on top of the mountain, and joy is in both the front row and the bleachers, if we are willing to be where we are. --- Mark Nepo

For those on journeys with cancer, I might paraphrase him by saying that light is in both the chemo IV bag and in the eyes of my compassionate nurse. Music is both in the deep, comforting voice of my oncologist as well as in the laughter of my grandchildren playing in the back yard even though I'm too ill to join them right now. Spirit is with me when I'm under the surgeon's knife and also when I am a year past the diagnosis and walking my dog on the beach. Joy is both in the cancer-me and the *healthy-me*, as long as I am willing to accept whatever place I am in.

Do you notice that the key here is a simple willingness to be where we are? For me, it's about acceptance instead of resistance. If I am struggling against the fact that I have to let go of several key work projects while I recover from surgery and chemo, then I won't be able to experience the benefits of simply resting for several hours each day, and the sheer luxury of an afternoon nap. If I am resisting the fact that I am dealing with cancer, then I'm probably going to miss the joy that comes when I notice the kindness of certain people who care for me.

Resistance takes up too much mental, physical and emotional energy. Acceptance of the journey allows us to be present with what is. And what is, is often joy.

You Try It! ~ Joy Points

I first heard of the idea of counting Joy Points while doing Emotional Brain Training (EBT) work with Laurel Mellin several years ago. The idea is to keep a running list and see if you can get up to 100 Joy Points in the course of a week. If it's Wednesday and you're already at 100, don't stop there! Keep counting. See how high you can go.

The big idea here is that *joy is in the little things.* Seeing a daffodil blooming on your trip to the library might incur a Joy Point for you. Noticing the warmth of the sun on your skin. Flowers sent to you from a friend. A greeting card that comes in the mail. A day when you don't have to take so many meds. Someone asking you how you're feeling. Good news from your surgeon (okay, that's not exactly a little thing!).

The other idea at work and play here is that *joy really is all around us* and all we have to do is pay attention. Be aware. Notice. It's not always easy to do this when we're climbing up the rocky cancer mountain, clinging with both hands and feet to keep from pitching off the metaphorical edge of the steep cliff. And yet. Here we are. Looking for the joy.

Here's one more thing to think about when it comes to the idea of Joy: *it's a choice.* We have to make a conscious decision to seek out the little (and big) Joy Moments of our lives, no matter what we are going through.

Wendell Berry said it best in these wise words:

Be joyful, though you've considered all the facts.

Take a look at what is happening in your life right now. The facts might not be pretty. The facts might well indeed be downright grim. No matter, decide right now that you are going to start counting Joy Points. Immediately. Not when you're feeling better or even later tonight. Now.

If you don't feel up to making a written list, keep the list going in your head until you have the energy to get out the pen and paper. Say "Joy Point!" in your mind whenever you notice that little (or big!) thing that makes your heart sing, even for a second. See if you can smile too. Every Joy Point counts. Every single one.

K is for... Kindness

I spent a lot of time in the Girl Scouts when I was growing up, and I learned to practice kindness there. We were encouraged to be kind to everyone, regardless of their color, culture, or physical appearance. I particularly remember working with mentally challenged children at a nearby hospital, and helping disabled teenagers at a summer camp. These powerful experiences of kindness followed me into adulthood.

When I was in my 30's, I began practicing yoga and that's where I learned the ancient practice of Metta, which is equal parts prayer and meditation. Metta focuses on loving-kindness... first to ourselves, then to those we love and who love us. After we are rooted in this love of self and community, we offer loving-kindness to those who bring us conflict, and finally to all sentient beings.

For the first part of my cancer journey, I was focused on the kindness that others were showing to me. The gentleness of my doctor's voice, the thoughtfulness of my brother and niece who came to visit me, the friend who left work early to sit with my husband while he waited for me to wake up from surgery, the cards and emails I received from people wishing me well. I actually chose *Kindness* as one of my four Anchor Words (see page 6-7) and it was a lovely mantra.

After I began to feel better, I remembered the prayer of Metta, and decided to add it to some of my morning meditation times. I found it to be rich and very rewarding.

It is important to me that the prayer begins by offering peace and kindness to *myself*. I hadn't really been doing that because, like most women, I'd been focusing on taking care of others, even during my cancer treatments. I found that once I shone the light of kindness on *me*, I was better able to offer it to others.

Metta has become an important way of life for me. As I write this, I'm in the middle of a disagreement with a good friend. She has greatly misinterpreted something that I wrote to her and now she refuses to speak with me about it. Instead of trying to make her wrong, I am giving her space, and I am trusting that when she is ready, she will reach out to me again. In the meantime, I offer myself kindness and I offer her kindness as well.

You Try It! ~ Metta

There is a lovely saying by Ian Maclaren:

Be kind for everyone is carrying a heavy burden.

Maybe you've heard this before. And you probably know this to be true. Everyone has a story they are living through and some of these stories are painful and difficult. The more kindness we can extend to others, the better we make the world. Agreed? Agreed!

HOWEVER.... I want you to focus right now, today, this moment (no putting it off any longer!) on extending kindness to *yourself*. If you're reading this book, then you must feel like *you* are carrying a heavy burden right now too. Start by offering yourself the same love, the same gentle kindness that you would show to any dear friend who is going through what you are going through.

1. Slowly say these words to yourself... and as you say the words, feel the warmth of your heart radiating towards all parts of your own being:

   May I be safe, May I be happy, May I be healthy, May I be free

Say it as many times as necessary until you feel a lightness in your body, mind and spirit.

2. Then hold your loved ones in your mind's eye, and say these words to yourself:

   May they be safe, May they be happy, May they be healthy, May they be free

3. In the last part of Metta practice, you can direct the energy of loving-kindness towards all sentient beings by slowly repeating these words to yourself:

   May all beings be safe, May all beings be happy,
   May all beings be healthy, May all beings be free

4. You might want to go back to Step 1 and repeat the loving-kindness mantra towards yourself.

L is for... Letting Go

In a beautiful short essay called "Welcome to Holland," Emily Perl Kingsley writes about what she had to let go of in order to welcome a disabled child into her life. She likens her journey to preparing for a trip to Italy. Imagine that you board the plane, which you think is heading to Italy. When the plane touches down, you are told "Welcome to Holland." *Say what?* You've planned your whole trip for *Italy*. Now, in a new country, you'll have to learn a new language, face new people and somehow, *somehow* let go of the original plan, which didn't have anything to do with Holland.

I can definitely relate to this. How about you? None of us were even remotely interested in planning a trip to The Land of Cancer. We were all in various orbits around various suns that had nothing to do with doctors, invasive tests, ugly hospital johnnies that pop open at all the wrong places, and sitting in recliner chairs with various colored drugs dripping into our veins while nurses scurry back and forth to monitor our blood pressure.

At some point on my journey, I had to *let go* of the resistance I was harboring towards this new path that had been thrust upon me. I had to say to myself in my own metaphorical jargon, "Welcome to Holland."

Within two weeks of my diagnosis in 2011, I had to let go of

1. a dear friend who died suddenly from a rare form of cancer
2. my best beloved 18-year-old cat Sasha who was having severe seizures
3. my left breast
4. The co-chair position of the SoulCollage® Facilitators' Conference that I'd been working on for two years

It all happened so fast, I hardly had time to process any of it until much later. I had to let go of a lot of things that summer of 2011. But the hardest thing to let go of was the knowledge that I was in a whole new metaphorical "country" that I had not chosen to be in.

What about you? What do *you* need to let go of today?

You Try It! ~ Both Sides Now

It is crucial for me to see that my life is not an *Either-Or* situation. For instance, when I say to myself "I hate having cancer," I am shutting off a whole new way of seeing things. I am relegating myself to a world that is black and white, end of story. But I can soften that statement by adding the word "and" to it, and completing it with something else that is also true. It sometimes takes me a while to figure out what that completing phrase might be, but that's okay. I have time!

Say this to yourself, out loud, right now: *I hate having cancer.*

Then say this, and see if you can feel a difference in your body, mind or spirit: *I hate having cancer AND I am grateful for my family and friends.*

You can turn anything harsh and critical around with this exercise. Take something that you don't like about yourself, add the word "and" and then add something else that is true about yourself that shows yourself in a more positive light.

For instance, *I am overly critical of my husband AND I love that we are planning a vacation together. I don't like how my body looks now that I've had surgery AND I am grateful for how my body has gotten me through everything so far. It totally sucks to be on this cancer journey AND I met a new friend in the waiting room the other day.*

"Both Sides Now" thinking opens up the possibilities for you to be able to enjoy bits of your life in spite of (or maybe even because of) the fact that you are dealing with cancer. It's something we're not conditioned to in our society. It's so much easier to complain and to get ourselves stuck in Either/Or thinking where there is only one way to think and feel and be.

Try this "Both Sides Now" exercise whenever you feel yourself sinking into the quicksand of negativity, fear and doubt. It's a surefire way to pop yourself right back up into the sunshine.

I am _____ AND _____.

I feel _____ AND _____.

I hate feeling _____ AND I like feeling _____.

M is for... Making Meaning

Discern the larger story in the midst of the everyday story.
Faith in life, or the process of change comes from finding meaning in your experience-
not THE meaning, as in "why is this happening to me?"-
but a sense that every experience will teach you something.
There are no mistakes, only growth opportunities.
Sense how you are being called to bring your gifts to the world through your challenges.
--- Jeanne Marie Merkel

What Jeanne Marie says here about discerning the "larger story" in the midst of our "everyday stories" is quite profound. If we can look at what is happening to us in our day-to-day experience with cancer (the blood tests, the bald head, the surgery, the treatments) in a way that embraces all that is larger than us, we can find a way to make meaning from our experience.

Throughout my life, I have continually challenged myself to take any difficulty that has crossed my path and find some kind of meaning in it. I was physically abused by my mother when I was 12. In my young adulthood I spent five years in an emotionally excruciating relationship with an alcoholic. The stepchildren I inherited when I married my husband in 1995 were angry and rebellious; I lost myself in their dramatic needs. I was treated for breast cancer in 2002. In 2004 my husband was diagnosed with prostate cancer and had to have extensive surgery. In 2008 he was declared legally blind from a rare genetic disorder. In 2011 I was diagnosed with secondary angiosarcoma of the same breast that was treated in 2002.

As you can see, I do have a lot of experience with "making meaning" when life doesn't go the way I want it to.

Now you're probably asking "*Just how exactly* do we do this?" In my own life I've found that the best way is by asking questions of myself. Writing/journaling works best for me, but you might find it suits you better to talk out your questions and answers with a loved one or therapist/guide instead.

You Try It! ~ Power of Questions

The work begins with questions. Asking a question can be a sacred act.
A real question assumes a dialogue, a link to the source from which answers come.
Questioning by its very nature is a spiritual practice.   ~ Susan Piver

Asking questions can be a deeply renewing spiritual practice. Hold this thought in mind while you work through the few questions suggested here. Living with these questions while you are on your cancer journey is a way to grow closer to Spirit (and yourself). It is a beautiful way to make meaning from any difficulties that life is throwing your way.

You could also use one or more of these questions to stay connected to your community of "others" by face-to-face and heart-to-heart discussions or phone conversations.

1. What do I believe is the "Larger Story" of the Universe? How did this Earth Planet come into being? What energy holds it in place? What faith or Being responds to me when I call out for help?

2. How can I let this Larger Story hold me during this challenging journey?

3. Have I found myself asking "Why me?" If so, try changing that question to "Why *not* me?"

4. Is there something that I can learn from my experience with cancer even though I didn't ask for it?

5. If there is something I can learn from this, how can I integrate this lesson into my life?

These questions are not meant to be answered immediately, nor all at once! I suggest that you print them out and look at them often. Allow the answers to come to you gently. Listen for the answers in your dreams, in your daily activities, in the stories that you read or see onscreen. Listen deeply wherever you are.

N is for... Now

The antidote to misery is to stay present. ~ Pema Chodron

I came across this quotation when I was in the midst of recovering from round after uncomfortable round of chemo. It was pretty much the last thing I wanted to hear, as you can imagine. Constantly tired, struggling with diarrhea and what I laughingly called "wonky stomach," I was not actually keen to "stay present" because I was so miserable. But as I thought more about this gentle suggestion, I realized that I *wasn't* staying present with the wonky stomach or the fatigue. I was trying *not* to be tired; I was wishing a thousand stars that I could eat whatever I wanted.

Another thing that continues to make me miserable (even though I'm 18 months past my last chemo treatment) is FEAR. Yes, the capital-letter kind of fear that invades my sanity and keeps me up at night. As you may have guessed, the cornerstones of this fear are: a) fear of the cancer coming back, and b) fear of dying young.

After many long months of living with this capital-lettered fear, I have discovered that truly, the only solution is to greet it kindly, "Hello Fear, there you are again." And then gently bring myself back to the present moment. I do this time and again by remembering to pay attention to my breath, which is a key element in bringing me back to Now.

One time after my first go-round with cancer and before the second, there was a suspect lump in my other breast. I found myself sitting in the surgeon's office for over an hour, waiting for test results. The fear was excruciating. The only thing that gave me peace and serenity was chanting this mantra over and over in my mind: *In this moment, I am safe.* Over and over and over. I even pulled out a little notebook that was in my purse and wrote it over and over. *Right now, in this moment, I am safe.*

I found that it was absolutely true. In that moment, I WAS safe! And I also realized that even if I got cancer again, I still would be safe. Moment to moment. *Right now.* Which is all I have, all I ever have.

I choose not to waste the precious NOW resisting what I am feeling.
I choose not to miss the joys of NOW by focusing on a fearful future.

You Try It! ~ Now Mantra

Find as many ways as you can to keep this mantra in the forefront of your daily activities:

In this moment, I am safe.

Here are some suggestions:

1. Print this page, cut out the mantra, glue it onto a piece of cardstock and prop it by your bed.

2. Use it as a bookmark.

3. Make it into a little song.

4. Write the words in your own handwriting on a big piece of poster board.

5. Find magazine images that represent "safety" to you and add them to the poster.

O is for... Open Heart

Stop the flow of your words,
open the window of your heart
and let the spirit speak.
~ **Rumi**

People of many different cultures believe that one's heart is the passageway between Father Sky and Mother Earth. In other words, the heart is not just an organ in the physical body. It is a spiritual place, an energetic space within each of us, a place that is not easily accessed with words, as Rumi states above. It is the place inside of us where Spirit speaks to us, where we speak to Spirit, and where we are united with the One Who Loves, the true Source of everything that exists.

So what does it mean to open our hearts, and what does opening our hearts have to do with creating a brighter and more meaningful cancer journey? Before we answer that, let's look at what it means to *close* our hearts.

Try this:

1. Stop reading for a moment and close one hand into a tight fist. Hold it while you slowly count to 10. Notice how it feels. Here are some words that came to mind when I did this just now: *tight, tense, stiff, painful, closed, rigid.* Can you add any words to that list? _____

2. Now, open that same fist, slowly uncurling your fingers one by one until your palm is exposed and your hand is once again relaxed. Here are some words that came to mind when I did this just now: *relief, gentle, free, easy, grace, relaxed.* Can you add any words to that list from your own experience? _____

For me, living from an open heart is something to practice, and not something I always do very well. It's a way of living from my center that feels freeing, easy, gentle and relaxed. I know immediately when I have closed my heart because my whole life begins to feel tense, rigid, stiff and tight.

If you're really listening, if you're awake to the poignant beauty of the world, your heart breaks regularly. In fact, your heart is made to break; its purpose is to burst open again and again so that it can hold evermore wonders. ~ Andrew Harvey

A little reminder before we begin this exercise: there are times when it's safer not to completely open our hearts. I repeat: *there are times when it's safer not to completely open our hearts.* For example, if a work colleague invites you for tea and only wants to talk about themselves or never asks you questions about what you are going through, you might not want to open your heart to this person. If there is someone in your life who has hurt or betrayed you, it's pretty safe to assume that you don't want to open your heart fully with them right now.

If someone or something (like cancer) has broken your heart, the tendency is to close down and stay closed down. But like Mr. Harvey says above, the heart is made to keep bursting open so it can hold more beauty, more connection, more wonders and grace and love. The trick is to find and connect with people who offer us safety, people who honor our open hearts with their own openness, acceptance and validation.

On the next page you will see 2 columns. The second column is headed with a rosebud that is closed up tight. Spend some time in the coming week making a thoughtful list in the **Closed Rose column** of people in your life whom you *don't* feel safe completely opening your heart to. Remember that it's perfectly okay to put people on this list you think you "should" be open-hearted with.

And at the same time, look around you for people you are already connected to who are holding your spirit in reverence, love and delight. *These* are the people it is safe and desirable to be open with. These are the people you can trust with your very precious heart. Put their beloved names on the **Open Rose list**. This list might include names of people you already know and connect with on a regular basis. But it can also include people in your life whom you intuitively trust even though you are not in relationship with them yet.

When you feel that your lists are complete (for now), sit back and take a look. Is one list longer than the other? Which one? If the Open Rose list is longer than the other, you are indeed very blessed! If your Closed Rose list is longer than the other, don't get down on yourself in any way…. It's ALL okay. All you need is ONE name on the Open Rose list and you are golden. If you don't have a name to put there, please feel free to put MY name there. I am happy to support you on this journey.

You Try It! ~ Open Rose/Closed Rose

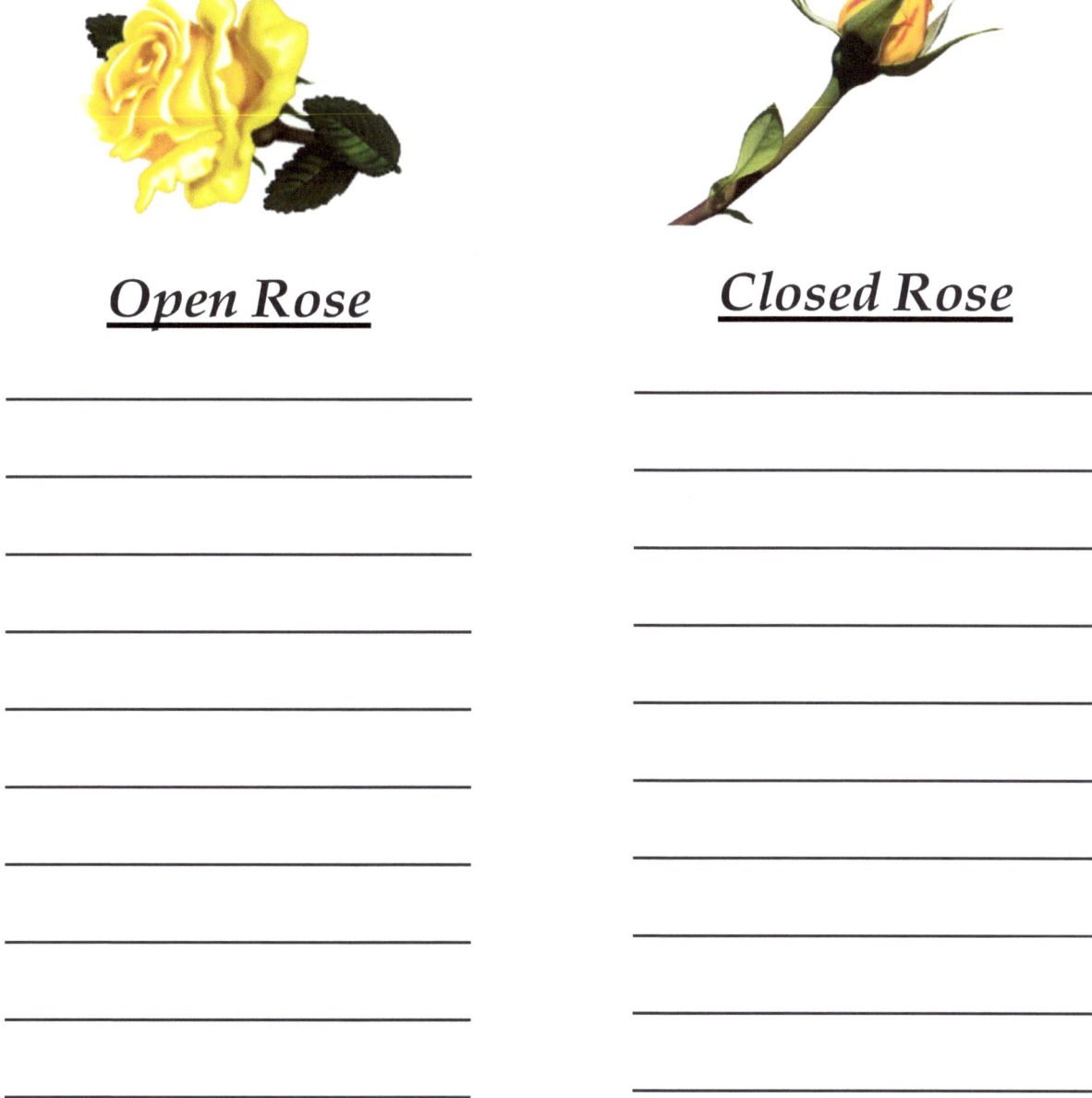

Open Rose

Closed Rose

_____

_____

_____

_____

_____

_____

_____

_____

P is for... Physical Body

Here in this body are the sacred rivers: here are the sun and moon
as well as all the pilgrimage places...
I have not encountered another temple as blissful as my own body.
---Saraha

Yes, our bodies are meant to be blissful temples, according to the Hindi poet Saraha. But it can be really hard to keep that in the forefront of our minds when we're lying flat on our backs with chemo drugs dripping into our veins or while trying to function under the lingering effects of anesthesia.

Even if we're turned inside out by the physical damages of cancer, it's important to hold in our thoughts that our body *does* contain sacred rivers, the sun, the moon, and places of pilgrimage. Every day, in some small way, it's crucial to stay connected to our physical bodies because they're just as important as our minds and spirits!

There are many ways to do this, and one of them is by becoming present to yourself through your breath. This is very simple, and you don't need to have any energy at all to practice it. Just close your eyes (if you're in a place where it's safe to do so) and listen to your breathing. Don't try to change it, just listen. Simply be with it.

Remember that you are a human being in a human body and be gentle with yourself.

Allow the breath to flow in and out. It might be smooth; it might be scattered. It might be full; it might be sparse. Just allow your breath to flow in and out.

A way to go deeper into your body with your breath is to mentally scan all of your body parts, starting at the top with your head, then moving down slowly, consciously paying attention to each place of your physical being- face, neck, shoulders, chest, back, stomach, arms, hands, legs, feet, toes. If you come across any tension or pain as you are scanning, consciously send light and breath (or a special color) into that place for a moment. See if you can be gentle with any anxiety or discomfort you feel in any part of your body.

You Try It! ~ Body Map

Don't go outside your house to see flowers.
My friend, don't bother with that excursion.
Inside your body there are flowers.   ~ Kabir

Take a large piece of poster board or drawing paper. Using a pencil, sketch an outline of your body. If you want to have more fun, lie on top of a huge sheet of paper and allow someone you love to trace the outline of your actual body using pencil, crayon or marker (in the colors of your choice, of course!).

Hang the outline where you can see it often, and when you feel up to it, start filling in the shape with color, paint, pictures, crayon, marker, or magazine pictures. You might want to fill it in with flowers, as Kabir suggests above.   Paint or draw swirls, polka dots, rainbows, magic rivers, sacred forests, flying giraffes, eagles' nests, dragonflies, or whatever has deep reverent meaning for *you*.

Keep this Body Map in a place where you'll see it often. Remember, it is only for you. You don't have to explain it to anyone else.

If you feel up to it, at some point you might want to say some gratitude prayers specifically for your body, for all that it is doing to keep you well and safe. You might not feel like doing it on some days, and that's okay. Just keep in the back of your mind that the more you offer gratitude to your beautiful body, the more it can offer you continuing strength and support on your journey.

At first, during my own Cancer Journey, it was difficult to think about this, much less say a prayer of gratitude about it! For a while, I thought that my body had betrayed me by forming cancer cells, and I wasn't in the right frame of mind to even think about offering it gratitude.

But the more I thought about it, the more I was able to say (and mean!) things like:

I am grateful to my body for being strong enough to survive the chemo treatments.
I am grateful to my legs for taking me for a walk outdoors today.
I am grateful to my eyes for continuing to allow me to see beauty.

How many parts of your body can you offer gratitude for today?

You Try It! – What Do I Need?

This exercise is similar to the one I describe in *F is for Flow of Feelings* (pages 17-19).

Instead of focusing on your emotions, try focusing on what your physical body is feeling. Use each sensation to determine what you need.

For example:

1. My head feels achy.
    I need to take a Tylenol and lie down in a dark room for 30 minutes.

2. My toes feel tingly.
    I need to call my doctor/nurse to ask what I should do.

3. My stomach feels empty but unwell.
    I need to eat some plain crackers and chicken broth.

4. I feel tired.
    I need to take a nap. OR I need to sit in the fresh air for five minutes and do nothing.

It sounds simple, right? It is… and yet sometimes it isn't. This leads me to another important part of this exercise. You have to give yourself PERMISSION to get what you need. It may be easy to recognize a headache but sometimes it's not so simple to give yourself permission to actually take the pill and let yourself lie down.

It might be a no brainer to know that your body is hungry but a bit more difficult to ask someone to heat up the soup and bring you the crackers.

On this cancer journey, a great deal of wisdom can be gained from giving yourself permission to take care of your whole self, *no matter what* that entails.

Q is for... Quiet Rest

*Sometimes the most urgent and vital thing you can possibly do
is take a complete rest. ~ Ashleigh Brilliant*

*Invite little pauses into your day,
spiritual catnaps that let your heart catch up with the rest of you.
~ Jennifer Louden, The Life Organizer*

One of the biggest blessings I received on my own cancer journeys was the ability to take time off from and greatly slow down my work. I know that not everyone has this luxury, but in my case, both times, I believe it greatly contributed to my healing. In 2002 I took five months off from my customer service job at the regional theatre where I'd worked for seven years. I had great big gobs of time to sleep, read, write in my journal and create art. Of course, a lot of that time, I didn't feel like writing or making art! But just the fact that I knew I had open-ended days was healing to me.

In 2011-12, my work revolved around my business KaleidoSoul.com. I was able to give some of the more basic tasks over to my fabulous assistant, Kate. Some of the work I dropped completely (giving workshops, leading Trainings). And the rest of it I was able to do at my own pace, whenever I felt like it.

Again, I know that I am extraordinarily blessed that I could do this. I was able to allow myself those "little pauses" and "spiritual catnaps" that Jennifer Louden speaks of above. I was able to lie down and nap whenever I felt like it. I was able to take comfort and peace in resting my physical body.

Whenever I was tempted to work instead of rest, I reminded myself of how much stress my body was going through. Surgery and/or any kind of cancer treatment puts an untold amount of strain on our bodies. The best medicine for that stress is quiet rest, and we must commit to giving that to ourselves whenever, wherever and however possible.

You Try It! ~ Boundaries

Boundaries are to protect life, not to limit pleasures.
~ Edwin Louis Cole

In order to give yourself the quiet rest that your body, mind and spirit need for healing, you need to decide that this is a priority, and then you need to put some boundaries in place in order to make it possible for it to happen.

For example, during my own healing from surgeries and chemo, I had to draw some boundaries with my husband's family. I had to be honest with myself. I had to really look at myself, my own personal needs and predilections, and then I had to stand up for myself. I did this by creating boundaries.

I had to say, "I'm not going to attend big family get-togethers until I am through this." And, "Please ask the kids not to come over for three days until I'm over the worst of this treatment."

Now your situation might be very different. My husband's children were not people that I found particularly nurturing; I didn't want to be around them when I was ill. I'm not a social butterfly on my best days; when I'm unwell, I find large gatherings hugely detrimental to my healing. Your boundaries are probably going to be different than mine, and that's okay. What's important is to start thinking about what *you* need in terms of quiet rest, and how you're going to give that to yourself. Once you have that in mind, you can focus in on creating boundaries.

Here are some questions to help you get started:

1. How much quiet rest do you need today?
2. How can you give this to yourself?
3. What boundary do you need to put in place to ensure that you get it?
4. Is there someone or something in your life that is making demands on you that you need to say "no" to?
5. What do these words from Brene Brown mean to you? *Daring to set boundaries is about having the courage to love ourselves, even when we risk disappointing others…. Only when we believe, deep down, that we* are *enough, can we say "Enough!"*

R is for... Reaching Out

Only connect.   --- E.M. Forster

One of the biggest parts of our S.O.S. mission is helping women with cancer stay connected to others. Self-connection and Spirit-connection is vitally important, yes. But we are not meant to be alone in this life. E.M. Forster had it right in what is the simplest, shortest quotation ever. We have only to *connect* to one other human being and our burden is lightened.

There is a wonderful African proverb that states: *If you want to travel swiftly, go alone. If you want to travel far, go together.* This is the purpose in seeking community of some sort while you are dealing with things like surgeries and uncertain outcomes and chemo treatments and trips back and forth to doctors that you may or may not enjoy visiting. You don't have to bear the load of this alone. Even though you can get through it all just fine by yourself, you'll find that you'll get farther with someone by your side who cares about you.

When I received my first diagnosis in 2001, I met two women on an internet support group for women with breast cancer. Dawn (in Missouri) was two months ahead of me on the same treatment path. Elizabeth (in Canada) was a whole year ahead of me. I was struggling with the question of *who to tell* about my diagnosis. Part of me wanted to not tell anyone except my husband, brothers, boss, and stepchildren. I have never been one to enjoy being the center of attention. I thought I would be on everyone's "pity list" if I told the people I worked with as well as all my friends and extended family.

Elizabeth told me that when she was first diagnosed, she had those same thoughts, yet she had consciously chosen to tell *everyone*. She was really glad she did because she had found support in unexpected places and she also found no support from people she had expected it from. So that is what I did: I told everyone, in the form of phone calls and emails. And the same thing happened to me. Two former bosses I'd lost touch with were there for me suddenly and our friendships were renewed. A few friends never replied to the email. A close friend who'd moved to the west coast took more than a month to call me and ask how I was.

But somehow, it all balanced out. I had just the right amounts of support at all the right times. It helped that when I sent the email, I let it go without expectations. I just put it out there and let it be.

I do have a confession to make. I was completely exhausted from the invasive tests prior to my diagnosis, from so many trips to the surgeon, and from talking about my treatment plan with my boss and people at work and my siblings. I didn't feel like I had enough energy to call my mother on the phone and tell her. I just didn't want to deal with her fear. Our relationship had been rough at times and I felt depleted just thinking about it. If I had been

53

doing the *Open Rose/Closed Rose* (see page 39) worksheet back then, my mother would have been on the Closed Rose list.

I told my husband Jeff that I had decided not to tell my mother until after the lumpectomy was over with, and he shook his head vehemently. "No, you have to tell her now," he said. I was surprised at this stand he was so staunchly taking. Up until then he had been with me by my side and quietly let me make all the decisions. When I told him I honestly didn't have the strength to tell her, he asked if I wanted him to call her instead and I agreed. He handled it well, and looking back on it, I'm glad that he did.

However, I would like to add here that it wouldn't have been the worst thing if he had not. We each have to make these decisions based on what is best for *us*, not on what is best for the others in our lives.

When I was diagnosed with secondary angiosarcoma in 2011, I was fortunate enough (still am!) to be connected to a worldwide community of SoulCollagers through my work as a SoulCollage® Facilitator and Trainer. I had hundreds of people on my KaleidoSoul email lists by then and I let everyone know what I was facing. The amount of support, prayers, love and positive energy that came to me from this community was nothing short of astounding. I literally, physically FELT the support in my body, mind and spirit throughout the ten months of surgeries and treatments.

Now, I'm not saying that YOU have to tell EVERYONE in YOUR life! I'm just saying that I did what felt right to me at the time. *We each have to make these decisions based on what is best for us, not on what is best for the others in our lives.* Find some quiet time with yourself and seek inner direction if this is a question that you are struggling with.

In the "You Try It" section on the next page, you'll find some suggestions for ways to reach out to others while you are on your cancer journey. Read them carefully. You don't have to do them all! Just try one or two that appeal to you right now.

You Try It! ~ Count the Ways

One of the most calming and powerful actions you can do to intervene in a stormy world is to stand up and show your soul. Struggling souls catch light from other souls who are fully lit and willing to show it. ~ Clarissa Pinkola Estes

Here are some suggestions for Reaching Out for support while you are journeying with cancer. Take what you like and leave the rest. Choose just one to try this week and see what happens!

1. Stop by our S.O.S. Cancer Journeys Facebook group and say hello. Tell us a little about yourself, no matter how you are feeling. It's a good, private place to check in and connect with other women who are journeying through cancer with grace, spirit and hope. This is a PRIVATE group, which means that none of your own Facebook friends can see what you are posting or read the other posts. *NOTE: If you are not on the group yet, click on the "Join Group" button near the top. If you can't find that button, just send me an email (annemarie@sos-cancer-journeys.com) and I will add you, no worries.*

2. Google search for other support groups online. The Facebook group above is for women with ANY kind of cancer, but you might find a support group focused on your kind of cancer more helpful. See what works for you!

3. Ask a friend or someone you work with to organize people to bring you (and your family) meals during the days immediately after surgery or treatments when you have the least energy. People really do want to help; they are just waiting to be shown what to do!

4. Write a letter, send an email, or call someone on your "Open Rose" list from the *Open Heart* section of this e-book (pages 37-39). Share any difficulties or challenges you are facing. Allow them to listen and love you through it, even if they don't have an immediate solution.

5. Send me an email and let me know how you are doing, or ask a question that's been simmering in your mind. annemarie@sos-cancer-journeys.com. Reach out. You are not meant to go through this alone!

S is for... Stories

I'm not saying that you should deny the difficult events of your life. But the fact that you survived is also a wonderful story to tell. And that story, the story of the way you came through a difficult situation, found resources within yourself or outside of yourself, gleaned from that experience what you wanted and what you didn't want going forward — that is a story that can inspire you and others to heal and grow.

~ Golda Poretsky

About three months after my final treatment for breast cancer in 2002, I attended a weekend retreat for Women Living with Breast Cancer at Kripalu Center for Yoga and Health in western Massachusetts. On the first morning of the retreat, the facilitator divided us into groups of four and we each had 30 minutes to tell our story to the other women in our group. I have to say, this was the most healing thing I experienced in my recovery from that entire cancer experience.

You might think that 30 minutes is too long, that you couldn't talk for half an hour to complete strangers about what you've been going through. But I would wager a bet that you'd be wrong! We were all a little nervous, of course, but once we realized we were in a safe, healing space with women who were actively listening to us, the words just flowed from our hearts to our lips. Tears also flowed but I assure you they were tears of healing, not tears of heartache!

There is a certain divinity in being truly listened to as we tell our stories. Miles Franklin said it best when he stated:

Someone to tell it to is one of the fundamental needs of human beings.

I wrote the entire story of my first cancer journey in my book *Bright Side of the Road: A Spiritual Journey Through Breast Cancer* which is still available on Amazon. In the writing of it, I did want others to benefit from my experience, but a greater motivation for me was the actual *telling of my story*. I needed the feeling of relief that comes, for me, from writing things out. It was a purging, if you will. Lots of feelings and thoughts were able to be digested and eliminated in the telling of my story, both at the retreat and in the book.

You Try It! ~ Tell Your Story

It is easy to be seduced by the idea that how things turn out is more important than what happens in the process. The real question is not, "How did it turn out?" The real question is "What happened to your spirit as you journeyed?" ~ Alan Cohen

There are several ways you can tell your own story. Here are some of them.

1. It's not necessary to speak for 30 minutes or to write an entire book in order to tell your story! Stop by our SOS Private Facebook Page and post a note to the group. If you don't feel up to writing a lot, just share your first name and where you're from and what kind of cancer you've been dealing with. That might be enough for now.

2. If you feel like writing about your story, try using any of these as starters:

   ➤ It all began when…
   ➤ Once upon a time…
   ➤ Now that I've been through cancer, this is what I know…
   ➤ I wish….
   ➤ Cancer is teaching me… or… Cancer has taught me….

3. If telling your story orally is more appealing to you, choose someone on your "Open Rose" list (in the *Open Heart* section, page 39) and ask if they will just listen to you while you talk about your Cancer Journey. Their job will not be to offer advice or suggestions, nor even to tell their own story (unless you agree to that ahead of time). Their job is only to listen nonjudgmentally and to hold your hand or offer you a tissue if you need one.

4. Try separating your journey into smaller parts, then writing about each one individually. Those pieces could include but are not limited to: Diagnosis, Surgeries, Radiation, Chemo, Doctors, Relationships, Lessons Learned.

If you would like some more support with the writing process, check out this very informative, supportive and helpful book: *When Words Heal: Writing Through Cancer, by Sharon Bray.*

Do not be satisfied with the stories that come before you.
Unfold your own myth.
~ Rumi

T is for... Time

Before my cancer diagnosis, I was living at an accelerated pace. My biggest priority was crossing as many things as possible off of my To-Do list every day. Then suddenly I had major surgery to face, and recovery from that surgery. Next came chemo treatments and another surgery after that. I was no longer physically or mentally able to live at such a fast pace. I found my To-Do lists growing shorter and shorter. Time slowed way down, to a slumbering crawl.

And I found that I actually *liked* it!

Don't get me wrong. I didn't like the surgeries or the chemo treatments themselves. But I found myself enjoying the time I'd been given to slow down. It was a huge relief, in some ways, to let go of my lengthy lists, and just allow my body to sink into rest and recovery. The burden of cramming as much as possible into every day was being eased from my shoulders and I liked the lightness that that brought to me.

Because of this slowing down of time for me, I found myself "listening inside" more often. Instead of relentlessly pursuing items on a checklist no matter how I was feeling, I let my IGS (Inner Guidance System) make the decisions for me. I was able to slow down enough to ask myself questions such as: *Does this really matter? Do I want to do this right now? What does my body need to be doing right now? What is a priority for me today?* Paying attention to my inner answers to these questions was a powerful healing step for me.

I found myself saying "no" to things that I used to do without thinking twice. For example, my husband's three children have given us eight glorious grandchildren ranging in age from newborn-11. When everyone gets together, it's a noisy and chaotic celebration of playful love. During my cancer recovery time, I chose not to attend these gatherings, even when they were in our own house! I felt much more comfortable seeing the kids and the grandkids one or two at a time instead of all at once. My energy felt less assaulted this way.

It might be very different for you. You might thrive during noisy family celebrations. This is where your own IGS comes in very handy. Get used to listening to yourself on the *inside* first.

You Try It! - Slow Time

The secret of life is enjoying the passage of time.
~ James Taylor

I am definitely NOT off my rocker when I suggest that you can slow yourself down enough to enjoy "the passage of time," even when you are journeying with or beyond cancer. Here are some suggestions:

1. If you continued to work through your treatments, take a few days off. Catch up on your reading or rent some movies you've been meaning to see. Take a nap in the middle of the afternoon. Heck, take a nap in the morning if you feel like it!

2. Make a list of things that you truly enjoy doing, whether or not you have the energy now to do all of them. Choose one thing that you *do* have energy for and find a way to do it today, right now!

3. Write in your journal about what the phrase "slow time" means to you.

4. Tune into your own IGS (Inner Guidance System) by allowing yourself a space of silence and stillness every day.

5. Allow your IGS to direct you towards saying no to something that doesn't feel "right" to you this week.

6. Write a real letter (with pen and pretty paper) to a friend instead of sending an email.

7. Look at this song lyric from James Taylor's *The Secret O' Life*, and spend some time thinking and journaling about how it feels for YOU.

Now the thing about time is that time
isn't really real.
It's just your point of view.
How does it feel for you?   ~James Taylor

U is for... U R Not Alone

I recently bought a smart phone and there are a couple of friends who regularly text with me, so I've learned the new "lingo" for abbreviating. We're getting near the end of the alphabet now and the word choices to explore are fewer and far between. So please allow me the liberty of abbreviation here when I emphatically state that *U R not alone.*

This is one of the biggest lessons I learned during my second cancer journey. If this is something you've already integrated into your beautiful life, please skip this section and move on to *V is for Viva La Gifts!* (pages 55-57). If not, please read on.

Since I was little, I have always enjoyed being alone. Reading, writing in my journal, and making up stories were all activities that I thrived on and I was happy being alone to do them. My siblings (two brothers) were older than me by 6 and 10 years, so my childhood was void of continual, close interactions with siblings. I kept one or two close friends throughout elementary and middle school and then found a close knit group of girls to hang out with in high school. Yet I never felt deprived. I actually blossomed and flourished, the more alone time I experienced.

As I grew into adulthood, I also grew into the shadow side of this love of being alone. When things got difficult, my solitude listed towards isolation. It was always difficult for me to reach out, to ask for help. Having seen my parents' and grandparents' old Yankee attitude of *I can do it myself, damn it* in action, I naturally grew up thinking that that's how difficult times were handled.

During my cancer journeys, however, it became very clear to me that I didn't *have* to "do it myself." I was able to see how many ways I was connected to so many people in my life. I realized that there were sources of assistance available to me in my community of friends and family, as well as spiritual guides and angels who surrounded me. My beloved cat Sasha died a week after my second diagnosis, and yet I was able to feel her presence and her singular love for me even afterwards.

I have discovered that the well of assistance available to us during any life crisis is deep and unending. All we have to do is believe that it is there, and then open to receive it.

You Try It! ~ Community Blessings Meditation

This activity is a listening one. You'll be guided inwards to a safe place of tranquility and beauty. Then your community members will join you in a large circle of support and comfort. You might be surprised by who shows up, so relax and allow whatever happens to happen!

In the years that I've been sharing this guided meditation, many people have told me that they weren't able to *see* anything, but they did *hear* something. Or they *felt* the environment with imaginary kinesthetic touch. Some of them just had a deep sense of knowing about something during the inner journey. All of this is perfectly okay!

Once in a while, someone doesn't see, hear, feel or imagine *anything*. That's perfectly okay as well. Certain inner journeys just don't "fit" with some people. And sometimes, a guided meditation needs to be listened to and experienced more than once in order to sufficiently relax and open up a person's inner world.

Give yourself permission to fall asleep. If that is what your body needs, you can allow it to happen. You can always listen to this meditation at another time as it's yours to keep and enjoy for always.

Listening time: 18 minutes

To listen online, click here:
http://www.audioacrobat.com/play/W0FfL82s

To download as an mp3 file, click here:

http://amber56.audioacrobat.com/download/cd189298-d39a-99b4-f938-e429ef72e6f0.mp3

When you are done listening, journal about the experience if that feels good to you, using the questions on the next page.

You might want to gather some photos or images of the people/animals who joined you in your Blessed Community Circle. Create a collage with them or place them somewhere you'll see them often. Use their names/photos as a reminder that you truly are NOT alone.

You Try It! ~
Community Blessings Journaling

These journaling questions were specifically designed to be used after listening to the Community Blessings meditation (page 53).

1. What safe place did you journey to? What memories does this place hold for you?

2. Describe how you felt when you were entering this place again in your imagination.

3. Make a list of the beings who joined you in this place, as many as you can remember:

   - From your current life

   - From your past

   - Those who have already passed over/transitioned

   - Pets, both past and present

   - Poets, artists, authors, actors, musicians, politicians… whom you've never met but whose work has touched your life

4. What did you feel when these beings were forming a circle around you? Was the predominant feeling Love? Fear? Gratitude? Sorrow? Joy? All of the above? Describe how you felt and what you were thinking as you watched them come in and beam love at you.

5. Did anyone show up who surprised you? Someone you'd forgotten, or someone who cares about you more than you thought? Who are they and why do you think they chose to be there with you today?

6. Did someone come forward with a special message for you? If so, who was it and what did they tell you or show you or give you?

7. How can this circle of community be helpful to you on your cancer journey right now?

8. Zora Neale Hurston said **Love makes your soul crawl out from its hiding place.** Did your own soul shine a little brighter while in the company of your blessed community circle? Has your cancer journey forced your soul underground in any way? In what ways did the loving imagery of this Magical Inner Journey help *your* soul come out of hiding, even the littlest bit?

V is for... Viva La Gifts

Is there any experience that you believe is outside of Spirit's plan for your good?
Can you reframe such an experience so you see it as a gift? ~ Alan Cohen

Alan Cohen is suggesting, in the above quote, that we *reframe* difficult situations and life challenges so that our focus is not on the *difficulty* but on the inherent *gift* instead. Believe me, this is not the easiest thing to do!

To "reframe" something means to take the general meaning and structure we've given to an event and *alter* it so that its shape is different in our minds. It's a conscious act; it's something that we deliberately *choose* to do. When *intention* blesses this act of reframing a difficult challenge, the gifts are made more clear to us.

Or, as one of my favorite teachers and guides likes to say to me when I encounter something unpleasant, "What can you learn from this?"

For me, that was the key question when it came to discovering what gift cancer had for me. Right after my second diagnosis, I wrote this in my journal as I flirted with the idea that cancer might have a gift for me:

This is a gift. It may not look like any other gift I've been given but it IS a gift. It is a Soul Lesson for me, but not just for me. It is a blessing to all those I am now serving and for all those I will serve in the future.

I still can't believe I wrote that, because at the time my mind was flooded with thoughts of preparing for a mastectomy and wondering if I would survive this aggressive angiosarcoma that was hibernating in my body. But I did write it, and I'm so glad I saved it. I'm glad I began, even early on, to look for the gifts in spite of the frustration, the anger, the fear, the difficult days ahead.

Rumi says:

The wound is the place where the light enters you.

Let us allow our own wounding to be lit by Spirit into a cornucopia of gifts.

65

You Try It! ~ Mandala of Gifts

I didn't begin working on this 18 x 18 Mandala until several months after my final surgery. And then once I started, it took me several months to complete it. I was running low on all kinds of energy (physical, creative, mental) after my 12 rounds of chemo and two surgeries, as you can well imagine.

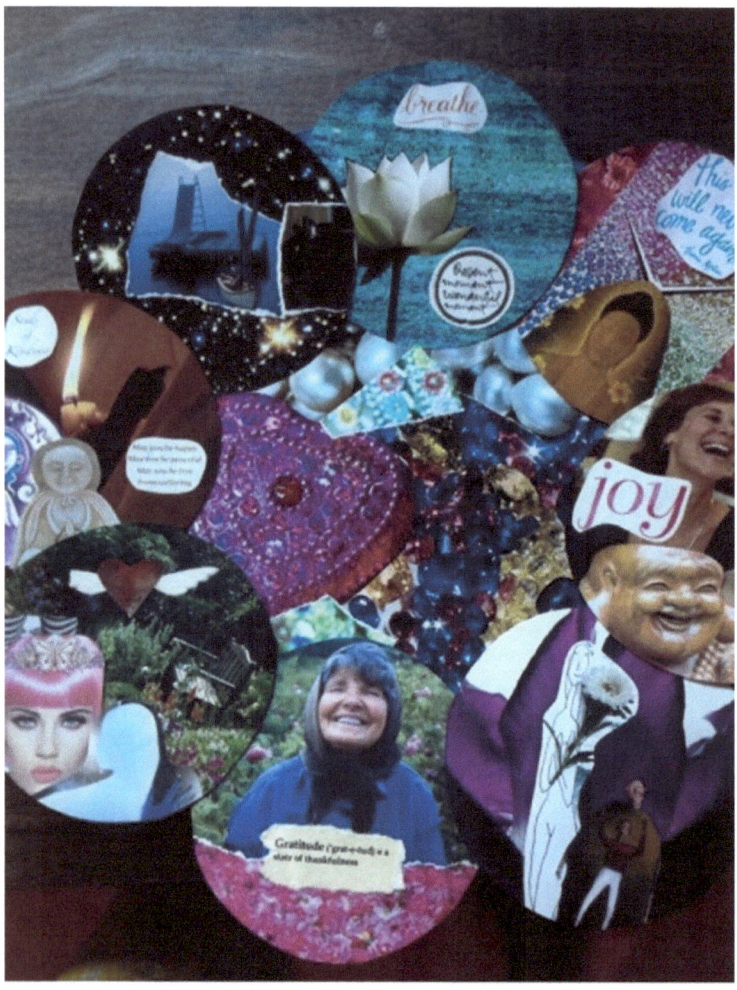

The word mandala means "circle" in Sanskrit and I used circular forms in this collage piece because I wanted the fluid feeling of wholeness and completion that circles give me.

The gifts reflected in this mandala are (starting at the top and moving clockwise, to the right):

1. Being in the present moment

2. Appreciation for today

3. Being open to joy

4. A strong, healthy body

5. Increased gratitude

6. Putting myself first

7. Kindness

8. Knowing that I am not alone

Instructions for creating your own Mandala of Gifts:

1. Spend some time journaling with these questions:

   ➢ What am I receiving on my Cancer Journey?
   ➢
   ➢ What am I learning?
   ➢ What do I want to take with me, going forward on my journey?
   ➢ If there are some gifts in this cancer experience, what are they?

   If you don't have a clue what to write about, or if you don't have the energy right now to do this journaling, that's okay! Just print the questions out and tape them on your mirror or set them on the kitchen table where you will see them often along the way. Sometimes we simply need to live with the mystery of the questions in order to discover the answers.

2. Choose 4-8 gifts that you have received from your cancer journey. Cut as many 5.5" circles from cardstock as you need.

3. Spend some time going through magazines and catalogs for images and words that reflect each gift. This might take a while! Remember, it took me several months to complete my own Mandala. Take your time.

4. Glue the images/words you've collected for each gift onto each of the cut-out circles.

5. Paint a large round paper mache circle with acrylic paints in colors that you love. This is optional. You don't have to paint the whole thing because it will all be covered except for the center.

6. Use tacky glue to glue each collage onto the round base. Choose the order intuitively. Remember, you are making this for *yourself*!

7. Glue embellishments onto or paint the center of the mandala in a way that is pleasing to you. I cut out words that say "Gifts From My Cancer Journey," but you can put anything there that you want!

8. Hang it the wall where you will see it often.

9. If you can, take a photo of it and post it on our private SOS Cancer Journeys Facebook page.

W is for... Words

I was born instinctively knowing the power of words to heal. I didn't see either of my parents or my two older brother writing their thoughts and dreams down on paper. I didn't see them making up stories or writing poems in spiral notebooks while sitting in the back yard watching the sun go down over the highway below. I did these things naturally and intuitively.

This tool of journaling, of expressing yourself with words, might not be something you are drawn to, or something that you've even attempted. However, I encourage you to give it a try and see what happens. You might not be led to continue journaling forever, but you might find some healing release with the exercises that follow.

One such exercise that I did before my chemo treatments started was to write a Love Letter to myself. I kept it in my journal which I wrote in a few times a week, and carried with me to read during each treatment session. It's amazing to me how these few paragraphs had the power to uplift me and keep me centered when I felt like I just couldn't stand it any longer.

Dear Anne Marie,

If you are getting discouraged from the side effects of these treatments, keep these truths in your mind and heart:

1. *It's not gonna last forever. In February you'll start feeling better and better and better.*
2. *This is a new and possibly exciting journey that you are on. Look at your new SoulCollage® cards. Let them speak to you. Nurture yourself with their wisdom.*
3. *The kinder and gentler you are to yourself, the easier it will be. Rest. Relax. You have permission to take time for yourself.*

Love always,
Your pre-chemo self

Now YOU try it. No matter what stage of the journey you're on, write a love letter to yourself. Remind yourself of who you really are. Keep the love letter where you'll read it often. Better yet, write yourself love letters often! You are your own best ally.

You Try It! ~
Spontaneous Writing

Spontaneous writing is also called stream of consciousness writing, free-intuitive writing, flow writing, free association, automatic writing, or intuitive writing. You can call it whatever you want because it's an excellent way to delve beneath your surface, rational thoughts.

So grab a notebook or a couple sheets of blank paper, along with your favorite pen or pencil, and get ready to begin!

Don't stop writing, don't think or cross out words, don't imagine what you'll write next or reread what you've written. Just move the pen, one word to the next. **If you feel stuck, keep your pen moving anyway.** You can make loops to keep going, or write your last word over and over again until the next thought and word appears. You don't have to use punctuation. You don't have to write in complete sentences. But you may. It doesn't matter. Nothing matters except to keep the pen moving. Go as fast or as slow as you want. Remember to breathe. And promise yourself that you are not going to judge yourself, whatever shows up on the page. No one is going to see your writing except YOU.

I am feeling…

I now see that…

I am ready to accept…

I believe…

I am…

I'm afraid that…

I love and appreciate…

The bright side is…

I want…

Maybe I can…

X is for... Xtra Self-Care

I might not need to remind you of this, but I'm going to anyway: now, more than any other time in your life, you need to give yourself Xtra Loving Care. The form that this takes for you will probably be different from any other woman with cancer, and that's okay. Once again, it's all about activating your IGS (Internal Guidance System), identifying what you personally need, and then finding a way to get it for yourself.

The first time I went through cancer, I had the lymph node dissection surgery under my left arm. Afterwards, I was told to be very careful with my left hand and arm because injuries there would be more susceptible to infection (because of the missing lymph nodes). Well, I'd been a nail biter since I was little, and I'd always *wanted* pretty nails. So I decided that a couple of times a month I was going to get a professional manicure complete with colorful polish. Simple and inexpensive, yes. But also priceless because it was a pleasure to look at my nails every day! An added bonus: I wasn't inclined to bite them anymore and I had lowered my risk of infection.

Other ways I practiced Xtra Self-Care during my Cancer Journeys:

- ❖ Let myself nap whenever I needed to.
- ❖ Cried when I felt like it.
- ❖ Got a monthly massage from a kind and gentle therapist.
- ❖ Watched all 10 seasons of Friends (made me laugh!).
- ❖ Got a pedicure now and then.
- ❖ Bought a beautiful wig that made me feel "normal" when I went out.
- ❖ Asked my friends and SoulCollage® community to send me snail mail instead of email.
- ❖ Enjoyed good novels from the library.
- ❖ Spent extra time sitting in my comfy chair with our cat Minnie on my lap.
- ❖ Took our dog Suzy to the dog park and watched her delight in running and playing with the other dogs.
- ❖ Shut the door to my study when I needed peace and quiet.
- ❖ Listened to guided meditations and affirmations on my way to sleep.
- ❖ Cuddled with my husband on the couch; asked for lots of hugs.

You Try It! ~ Pampering

This is not the kind of activity where I can tell you what to do! This one is going to take a lot of inner sleuthing on your part. Basically, it comes down to asking yourself these questions:

1. What do I need?
2. What will make me happy?
3. What gives me pleasure and delight?
4. How can I take care of my body? What does it need right now? What feels good?
5. How can I take care of my mind today? Does my brain need stimulation or rest?
6. How can I take care of my spirit? What does my soul need right now? How can I connect with Spirit (or whatever you choose to call Spirit) today?
7. What would be soothing to me?

Before we leave this topic, I want to talk about food. It's vitally important that we listen to the *body* and not the *mind* when it comes to our eating. There are foods that keep our bodies strong and healthy, but these foods are different for each person. You can read every book on nutrition and cancer that there is, but when you're sitting at the dinner table, only *you* and only *your* body can tell you what to eat or not eat.

For instance, I knew that vegetables and fruit and other high fiber foods are recommended for cancer patients. But when the kind of chemo I was receiving met *my* particular stomach, it became apparent that I wasn't going to be eating very much of that at all! During the four months that I went through chemo, I had to stick to plain and simple foods with very little fiber to avoid diarrhea and all kinds of stomach problems. At first I was discouraged and upset about this, because I wanted to be eating "healthy." It turned out that what *was* healthy for me during my chemo was just about zero fiber and absolutely no dairy. I finally came to accept this, and chose to care for myself by choosing foods that worked for my body at that particular time.

So when you are looking at giving yourself heaps of Xtra Self-Care during your cancer journey, be sure to take a look at how you are feeding your body and what your body needs.

Y is for...
You Are Not Your Cancer

Reclaim your identity!
Remember that before you were a mother,
daughter, grandmother, teacher,
wife, artist, or corporate executive...
Before you were overweight, a recovering addict,
cancer patient, or incest survivor...
you were a powerful, spiritual being of light...
and that is who you shall be forever more.
Remind yourself of this daily...
hourly, if necessary...
and your life will transform
in powerful, positive ways.
~The Little Book of Light, by Mikaela Jones

I am so passionate about this topic! If I could have figured out a way to fit this one at the very beginning of this book, I would have. But Y comes at the end of the alphabet. I hope you take to heart what I'm going to say here. It is crucially important to journeying with cancer in a way that keeps us connected to Self, Others, and Spirit.

No matter what kind of cancer experience you've been through, no matter how long you've been going through it, no matter how difficult it is... it is not YOU. It is just a part of your life story. It is just something that you are going through for now.

In my book *Bright Side of the Road*, I share how I came to this conclusion. I'd been thinking and fretting and worrying all week after I was diagnosed. So much to think about. So many decisions to make. I was sitting in my office at the theatre where I worked, entering patron subscription data into the computer and my eyes rested for a while on the sun setting over the trees beyond my window. This thought just came to me and rested in my mind, offering comfort and strength: *I have cancer and I'm going to survive it.*
It's not going to kill me; it's just going to be one more interesting thing about me.

In the activity that follows, take your time. Try to relay this very important information to your body and spirit as well as your mind. **You are not just a cancer patient. You are special, uniquely beloved in all the world, a powerful spiritual being of light.**

You Try It!~ One More Interesting Thing

Getting sick is something we experience- it's not who we are. Although it's a part of us, it doesn't define us. ~ Tieraona Low Dog, M.D., Life is Your Best Medicine

Below is a numbered list. Next to #10, write something like "I have _____ cancer." Or "I had _____ cancer _____ years ago." Then, fill in the other lines above it with other interesting things about you. My list includes things like "My guiltiest pleasure is American Idol," "I once spent a whole week without talking at a meditation retreat," "I am passionate about theatre," "My pets are like family to me," and "I'm good at making collages." What will YOUR list say?

There is no magic to the number 10. Your list might have 6 things, or 7 or 22. Just play around with it. Allow this activity to remind you that there is much more to you than being a cancer patient!

1.

2.

3.

4.

5.

6.

7.

8.

9.

10.

Z is for...

Zebra & Other Animals

You know, people come to therapy really for blessing.
Not so much to fix what's broken as to get what's broken blessed.
In many cultures animals do the blessing because they are the divinities.

~ James Hillman

This section is about allowing animals to bless us. If you have pets of your own, you probably already intuitively understand exactly how animals offer us grace and blessing. My own cats, Sasha and Scooter were devoted companions to me the first time I went through cancer treatments in 2002. In 2011-12, they were both with me in spirit, and our dog Suzy and cat Minnie took their physical place at my side (and on my lap!).

But even if you don't have pets, you can still benefit from the blessings of animals by using your imagination and the guided imagery meditation on the following page.

You might not need to listen to the meditation, though. You might already have a sense of an animal guide (also called totems or companions) who is watching over you, protecting you, leading you on your journey. I have a friend who has been drawn to white tigers since she was little, and another who collects leopards. I don't have an affinity towards either of those animals but I am inexplicably drawn to Dolphin, Sea Lion and Dragonfly, to name a few.

You Try It! ~
Circle of Animals Meditation

Try to think of Animal Guides as imaginary companions on your journey. I can tell you from my own experience that they may *seem* imaginary, but their energy is very real.

By observing how each animal lived, found mates, located food and protected itself, Native Americans were able to define an animal's particular strengths and weaknesses. For example, bears hibernated during the winter, so it was said that they possessed the magic of dreams. They were also formidable foes, so Bear Energy was also about physical power and strength. It's fascinating to note that different cultures (not just Native Americans) came up with similar interpretations for individual animals.

Animal Guides also make themselves known to us in dreams. Pay attention to any animals that show up in your nighttime meanderings. Also notice animals in your day-to-day life. Are you seeing Spider everywhere? Has Crow suddenly made an appearance in your neighborhood? Is Chipmunk paying you daily visits in your backyard?

Another way to discover your personal Animal Guides is through the art and process of SoulCollage® as created by Seena B. Frost. You might find her book, *SoulCollage® Evolving*, helpful, as well as her CD: *The Companions Suit* which has more information about Animal Guides on it.

It is important to honor our Animal Guides, no matter how they make themselves known to us. One way to honor them is to pay attention to what they have to say to us. You can do this by using this guided meditation (Magical Inner Journey) or by journaling imaginary dialogues with them. Be sure to ask your Animal Guide(s) for wisdom about your own Cancer Journey.

To listen online, click here:
http://www.audioacrobat.com/play/Wd1pyRZs

To download as an MP3 file, click here:
http://amber56.audioacrobat.com/download/1bc7f362-31cd-e673-8a7f-ee4918e1acdc.mp3

Did you enjoy this Book?

If so, it makes my heart happy!

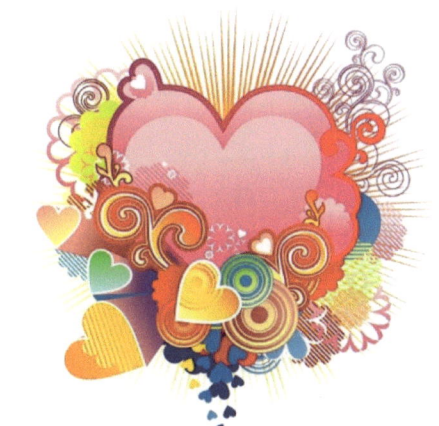

I am grateful to you for purchasing this workbook. My hope
is that you have received something positive from it, and that it makes your cancer journey a
bit lighter, easier, or brighter in some way.

**If this book was helpful to you and you think it might help someone else, please encourage
your friends, family and colleagues to download it for themselves here:**
http://sos-cancer-journeys.com/sunflower-spirit

I gladly welcome any comments, questions or feedback you'd like to share with me about this
e-book, the S.O.S. website, and/or about your own journey.

Please email me: annemarie@sos-cancer-journeys.com **or join us on our private Facebook
Group**: https://www.facebook.com/groups/457988474238141/

Also, be sure to **subscribe to our free monthly newsletter**, *Still Life with Cancer* for more
inspiration and support for your journey.   www.sos-cancer-journeys.com/still-life

I send you blessings and peace for a continuing journey of health, wellness and deeper
connection to Self, Others, and Spirit.

Much peace and joy in this moment,

Anne Marie Bennett

Anne Marie Bennett
PO Box 745
Beverly MA 01

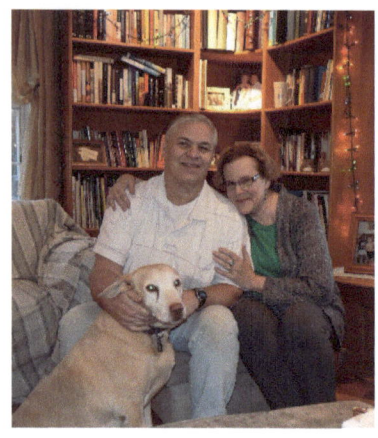

About the Author

Anne Marie Bennett is a writer, self-taught artist, website goddess, two-time cancer survivor, and SoulCollage® Facilitator Trainer who was mentored directly by Seena Frost, the creator of SoulCollage®. She has also worked as a bookseller, sheet presser, library assistant, second grade teacher, educational computer consultant, and in theatre management.

Anne Marie is the creator of SOS Cancer Journeys, a website that offers support, community and encouragement to cancer patients/survivors. She has been leading creative personal growth workshops and retreats since 1985 and is a published author and artist. Her workshop participants flourish as she gently guides them through the process of self-discovery while encouraging playful, creative self-expression with a joyful open heart.

Anne Marie has reached thousands of people with her positive message about the power of staying connected to Self, Others and Spirit when dealing with cancer. She is passionate about bringing this message to as many people as possible.

She grew up in Connecticut, graduated from Southern Connecticut State University and taught second grade for six years in Virginia. Anne Marie now lives, laughs, sings, writes, and creates art in eastern Massachusetts with her husband Jeff and their much loved yellow lab Suzy.

You can reach her at SOS-Cancer-Journeys.com.